FOREIGN TRAVEL & IMMUNIZATION GUIDE

12th Edition

Hans H. Neumann, MD

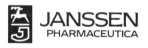
Medical Economics Books
Oradell, New Jersey 07649

Library of Congress Cataloging in Publication Data

Neumann, Hans H.
  Foreign travel & immunization guide.

Oradell, N.J., Medical Economics Co. Inc.

  Key title: Foreign travel & immunization guide, ISSN 0193-0338.

  1. Immunization—Handbooks, manuals, etc. 2. Travel—Hygienic aspects—Handbooks, manuals, etc.   I. Title.

RA638.N48   614.4'7'0202   79-640996

Design by Elaine Kilcullen

ISBN 0-87489-466-2

Medical Economics Company Inc.
Oradell, New Jersey 07649

Printed in the United States of America

CONTENTS

HOW TO USE THIS GUIDE

Find in the Index of Countries the page number for each country the traveler plans to visit, however briefly, and refer to the pages that apply. Don't include short stopovers when the traveler won't be leaving the airport.

Sections I and II are addressed chiefly to health-care providers. Section III contains health-related recommendations for the traveler.

PUBLISHER'S NOTES

If ever there were a perfect match of author to subject, it would be Hans H. Neumann and his "Foreign Travel & Immunization Guide."

Since the receipt of his medical degree in Vienna, Dr. Neumann's primary professional interest has been in the area of public health, with emphasis on preventive medicine. His research has taken him to countries on all the continents. He spent four years with the New Zealand Public Health Service working in the South Pacific and has done research in East and West Africa, in the Amazon Valley of Peru, and in East Asia.

While in private practice in the New York City metropolitan area, Dr. Neumann also served for many years as a research associate on public health projects at Columbia College of Physicians and Surgeons. Subsequently, for 17 years, he was Director of Preventive Medicine for the New Haven, Connecticut, Department of Health.

PREFACE

While immunization requirements for international travel have been eased in recent years, there is an increased need to follow recommendations that go beyond what is required. Malaria is spreading and chloroquine-resistant malaria organisms have become widely prevalent. More travelers are returning from abroad with malaria, infectious hepatitis, and parasitic diseases.

The good news is that no new cases of smallpox have been seen for many years, making immunization against it obsolete.

Not every immunization listed here as "required" is a strict legal requirement of the named country. Such "required" designations also include the probable requirements on arrival at subsequent destinations after visiting a potentially infected zone. Travelers should be prepared for immunization demands that various countries may impose, even if their rationale isn't evident.

Recommendations cannot be standardized. An anthropologist or geologist "roughing it" in a remote area faces different risks than those of a businessman staying in a luxury hotel in a city.

This guide is based on data from the World Health Organization, the Centers for Disease Control, and sources within the countries themselves, as well as my personal experience.

Hans H. Neumann, MD

I
IMMUNIZATION REQUIREMENTS AND RECOMMENDATIONS, BY COUNTRY

Austria	Gibraltar	Portugal*
Belgium	Great Britain	Romania
Bulgaria	Greenland	Russia
Canada	Hungary	Spain
Czechoslovakia	Iceland	Sweden
Denmark	Ireland	Switzerland
England	Italy	Turkey*
Finland	Luxembourg	U.S.A.
France	Netherlands	U.S.S.R.
Germany (East)	Norway	Yugoslavia
Germany (West)	Poland	

There are no immunization requirements to enter these countries from anywhere.

Recommended: Tetanus booster in last 10 years

*high risk of diarrhea

Albania	Greece	Malta

No immunization requirements, except for travelers who enter from tropical Africa or South America. Follow the requirements and recommendations for all countries on the itinerary.

Malta may require cholera immunization on arrival from tropical Africa or Asia.

Recommended: Tetanus booster in last 10 years

Bermuda	Cyprus	St. Helena
Canary Is.	Dominican Rep.	St. Pierre,
Cayman Is.	Falkland Is.	Miquelon
Cuba	Puerto Rico	Virgin Is.
		(British, U.S.)

No immunization requirements for travelers.

Recommended: Tetanus booster in last 10 years
Polio immunization up to date

Antigua	Dominica	Reunion
Aruba	Grenada	St. Kitts
Azores	Guadeloupe	St. Lucia
Bahamas	Jamaica	St. Martin
Barbados	Madeira	St. Vincent
Barbuda	Martinique	Tobago
Cape Verde Is.	Mauritius	Trinidad
Curacao	Netherl. Antilles	

No immunizations requirements except for travelers arriving from tropical Africa or South America. Follow the requirements and recommendation for all countries on the itinerary regarding yellow fever and other immunizations.

Cape Verde may require cholera immunization on arrival from a tropical African country.

Recommended: Tetanus booster in last 10 years
Polio immunization up to date

Mexico*

No immunization requirements, except:

Required: Yellow fever, on arrival from Bolivia, Brazil, Colombia, Peru, and from tropical African countries. Follow the requirements and recommendations for all countries on the itinerary.

Recommended: Typhoid and immune globulin (not needed if caution is used in the selection of food and eating places) Tetanus booster in last 10 years Polio immunization up to date Malaria pills (Chloroquine) recommended for southern regions and Yucatan. (Not needed for brief visits to cities.) Travelers to resorts on either coast (malaria risk low); use general precautions. After sunset:
1) stay in screened-in areas
2) use insect repellent sprays
3) avoid scented soaps and lotions
4) wear light colored clothing with long sleeves and long trouser legs.

For additional precautions regarding food and drink, and malaria, see Section III.

*high risk of diarrhea

Belize*	Guatemala*	Nicaragua*
Costa Rica*	Haiti*	Paraguay*
El Salvador*	Honduras*	

No immunization requirements for arrivals from the U.S., Canada, or Europe.

Required: Yellow fever on arrival from Bolivia, Brazil, Colombia, Peru, and from tropical African countries. Follow requirements and recommendations for all countries on the itinerary regarding yellow fever. (Yellow fever immunization—not required by Costa Rica.)

Recommended: Typhoid and immune globulin (not essential if caution can be used in the selection of food and eating places)
Tetanus booster in last 10 years
Polio immunization up to date
Malaria pills (Chloroquine): not needed for visits limited to cities; in Haiti recommended also for urban areas.

*high risk of diarrhea

French Guiana*   Guyana*   Suriname*

Required or strongly recommended: Yellow fever
Recommended: Typhoid and immune globulin
      (particularly for rural areas)
      Tetanus booster in last 10 years
      Polio immunization up to date
      Malaria pills (Chloroquine); also carry
      Fansidar, unless sensitive to sulfa drugs
Malaria risk exists, except in urban areas of Guyana and Suriname. See "Malaria" in Section II and III.

Brazil*   Panama*   Venezuela*

There are no immunization requirements for direct travel to and from the U.S., Canada, or Europe.
Required: Yellow fever, depending on subsequent
      destination. Follow requirements and
      recommendations for all countries on
      itinerary.
Recommended: Typhoid and immune globulin
      (not for visits limited to cities and
      resorts)
      Yellow fever (for visits to non-urban
      areas)
      Tetanus booster in last 10 years
      Polio immunization up to date
      Malaria pills (Chloroquine); also carry
      Fansidar, unless sensitive to sulfa drugs
Malaria risk: in rural areas and in the entire Amazon basin. See "Malaria" in section II and III.

Bolivia*   Ecuador*
Colombia*   Peru*

There are no immunization requirements for direct travel to and from the U.S., Canada, or Europe.

Required: Yellow fever, if a subsequent destination is a Caribbean island, a Central or South American country, Mexico, Africa, or Australia. Follow requirements and recommendations for all countries on itinerary.

Strongly recommended: Yellow fever, for visits to non-urban areas.

Recommended: Typhoid and immune globulin (for rural areas)
Tetanus booster in last 10 years
Polio immunization up to date
Malaria pills (Chloroquine), except for visits limited to major cities; also carry Fansidar, unless sensitive to sulfa drugs

See "Malaria" in section II and III.

Argentina*   Chile*   Uruguay*

There are no immunization requirements for arrivals from anywhere.

Recommended: Tetanus booster in last 10 years

*high risk of diarrhea

Algeria*   Libya*   Tunisia*

There are no immunization requirements for travelers, except:

Required: Yellow fever on arrival from tropical African and South American countries. Follow requirements and recommendations for all countries on itinerary.

Recommended: Typhoid and immune globulin (not needed if caution can be used in the selection of food and eating places)
Tetanus booster in last 10 years
Polio immunization up to date

Malaria risk: minimal. No malaria in most areas.

Israel   Jordan*   Kuwait   Morocco*

No immunization requirements for travelers.

Recommended: Tetanus booster in last 10 years

Egypt*   Iran*   Lebanon   Syria*

No immunization requirements for international travelers, except:

Required: Yellow fever on arrival from tropical African and South American countries. Follow requirements and recommendations for all countries on itinerary.

Recommended: Typhoid and immune globulin
Cholera for Iran
Tetanus booster in last 10 years
Malaria pills (Chloroquine) for rural areas

Malaria risk from May to October in rural areas, including the upper Nile Valley.

*high risk of diarrhea

Bahrein*	Qatar*	Yemen*
Iraq*	Saudi Arabia*	Yemen,*
Oman*	Arab Emirates*	Democr.

No immunization requirements for international travelers, except:

Required: Yellow fever for arrivals from tropical African and South American countries. Follow requirements and recommendations for all countries on itinerary.

Recommended: Typhoid and immune globulin (not essential if caution can be used in the selection of food and eating places) Tetanus booster in last 10 years Polio immunization up to date Malaria pills (Chloroquine)

Malaria risk in most areas except in cities.

No risk in Bahrein and Qatar.

Afghanistan[*]   Bangladesh[*]   Pakistan[*]

No immunization requirements for international travelers, except:

Required: Yellow fever, on arrival from tropical African and South American countries (see other countries on itinerary).
Cholera (for Pakistan), on arrival from infected areas: follow requirements and recommendations for all countries on itinerary.

Recommended: Malaria pills (Chloroquine)
Malaria risk present in all areas
Typhoid, immune globulin
Tetanus booster in last 10 years
Polio immunization up to date

[*]high risk of diarrhea

India*   Laos*
Kampuchea*   Vietnam*
(Cambodia)

No immunization requirements for international travelers, except:

Required: Yellow fever, on arrival from tropical African and South American countries. Follow recommendations for all countries on itinerary.
Cholera, if subsequent itinerary includes Pakistan, Malta, or an African country.

Recommended: Typhoid,
Immune globulin
Tetanus booster within last 10 years
Polio immunization up to date
Malaria pills (Chloroquine); also carry Fansidar, unless sensitive to sulfa drugs

Malaria risk in all areas.

See "Malaria" in Section II and III.

Burma*   Malaysia*
Indonesia*   Thailand*

No immunization requirements for international travelers, except:

Required: Yellow fever, on arrival from tropical African and South American countries. See requirements and recommendations for other countries on itinerary.

Required or strongly recommended: Cholera, if the subsequent itinerary includes Pakistan, Malta, or an African country

Recommended: Typhoid
Immune globulin
Tetanus booster in last 10 years
Polio immunization up to date
Malaria pills (Chloroquine); also carry Fansidar, unless sensitive to sulfa drugs.

Malaria risk in non-urban areas.

See "Malaria" in section II and III.

*high risk of diarrhea

Bhutan*   Nepal*
Maldives*   Sri Lanka*

No immunization requirements for international travelers, except:

Required: Yellow fever, on arrival from tropical African or South American countries (see these).

Recommended:
Typhoid
Immune globulin
Tetanus booster in last 10 years
Polio immunization up to date
Malaria pills (Chloroquine)

Malaria risk in rural areas.

Brunei*   Singapore   Taiwan

No immunization requirements for international travelers, except:

Required: Yellow fever, on arrival from tropical African or South American countries (see these).

Recommended: Tetanus booster in last 10 years
Polio immunization up to date

China   Philippines*

No immunization requirements for international travelers, except:

Required: Yellow fever, on arrival from tropical African or South American countries. (See requirements and recommendations for all countries on itinerary.)

Recommended: Typhoid
Immune globulin
Tetanus booster in last 10 years
Polio immunization up to date
Malaria pills (Chloroquine); also carry Fansidar, unless sensitive to sulfa drugs

Malaria risk in some rural areas, not in cities.

See "Malaria" in sections II and III.

Hong Kong   Korea (South, North)   Mongolia*
Japan   Macao   Seychelles

No immunization requirements for travelers.

Recommended: Tetanus booster in last 10 years
Polio immunization up to date

*high risk of diarrhea

Djibouti*   Ethiopia*   Somalia*

Recommended:
> Cholera (for Somalia)
> Yellow fever
> Typhoid
> Immune globulin
> Tetanus booster within last 10 years
> Polio immunization up to date
> Malaria pills (Chloroquine)

Malaria risk, except in Ethiopian highlands and in Addis Ababa.

Burundi*   Rwanda*   Tanzania*
Kenya*   Sudan*   Uganda*

Recommended:
> Yellow fever
> Typhoid
> Immune globulin
> Cholera
> Tetanus booster in last 10 years
> Polio immunization up to date
> Malaria pills (Chloroquine); also carry Fansidar, unless sensitive to sulfa drugs

Drug resistance widespread.

See "Malaria" in Sections II and III.

Central Afr. Republ.*	Ghana*	Niger*
Gabon*	Guinea-Bissau*	Nigeria*
Gambia*	Liberia*	Senegal*
	Mauritania*	Togo*

Required or strongly recommended: Yellow fever

Recommended:
>Typhoid
>Immune globulin
>Cholera
>Tetanus booster in last 10 years
>Polio immunization up to date
>Malaria pills (Chloroquine); also carry Fansidar, unless sensitive to sulfa drugs

Malaria risk high; drug resistance is spreading in West Africa.

See "Malaria" in Sections II and III.

*high risk of diarrhea

Angola*	Congo*	Mali*
Benin*	Equatorial	Sao Tome*
Burkina Faso*	Guinea*	Sierra Leone*
Cameroon*	Guinea*	Zaire*
Chad*	Ivory Coast*	

Required or strongly recommended: Yellow fever

Recommended:
> Cholera
> Typhoid
> Immune globulin
> Tetanus booster in last 10 years
> Polio immunization up to date
> Malaria pills (Chloroquine); also carry Fansidar, unless sensitive to sulfa drugs

Malaria risk high; drug resistance spreading in West Africa.

See "Malaria" in Sections II and III.

Comoro Is.*   Mozambique*   Zambia*
Madagascar*   Namibia*   Zimbabwe*
Malawi*   Swaziland

Required: Yellow fever on arrival from a tropical African or South American country. Follow requirements and recommendations for all countries on itinerary.

Recommended:
Cholera for Madagascar, Mozambique, and Swaziland
Typhoid
Immune globulin
Tetanus booster within last 10 years
Polio immunization up to date
Malaria pills (Chloroquine); also carry Fansidar, unless sensitive to sulfa drugs

Malaria risk and drug resistance in most areas. In Zimbabwe, no risk in city of Harare.

See "Malaria" in Sections II and III.

*high risk of diarrhea

Botswana*   Lesotho   South Africa

Required: Yellow fever on arrival from a tropical African or South American country. Follow requirements and recommendations for all countries on itinerary.

Recommended:

Typhoid (for rural areas)
Immune globulin (for rural areas)
Cholera for Lesotho, on arrival from a tropical African country
Tetanus booster in last 10 years
Polio immunization up to date
Malaria pills (Chloroquine)

Malaria risk limited to northern rural areas of South Africa and of Botswana.

Christmas Is.	Nauru	Samoa
Cook Is.	New Caledonia	(Western)
Fiji	Niue	Tahiti
French	Pacific Is, U.S.	Tonga
Polynesia	Trust	Tuvalu
Guam	Pitcairn Is.	Wake Is.
Kiribati	Samoa	
(Gilbert)	(American)	

No immunization requirements for arrivals from the U.S., Canada, other Pacific islands, Australia, and New Zealand.

For arrivals from other countries, follow the requirements and recommendations for those countries.

Recommended:

> Typhoid (not needed if caution is used in the selection of food and eating places)
> Tetanus booster in last 10 years
> Polio immunization up to date

Malaria risk: none.

Australia　　　New Zealand

There are no requirements for travel between the U.S., or Canada and Australia, New Zealand, and the South Pacific Islands en route.

For arrivals from other countries, follow the requirements and recommendations for those countries.

Recommended: Tetanus booster in last 10 years

Papua-　　　Solomon Is.*　　Vanuatu*
　New Guinea*　　　　　　　　(New Hebrides)

There are no immunization requirements if the previous two weeks were spent in Australia, New Zealand, other South Pacific islands, the U.S., or Canada.

For arrivals from other countries, follow the requirements and recommendations for those countries.

Recommended:
　　　　Typhoid
　　　　Immune globulin
　　　　Tetanus booster in last 10 years
　　　　Polio immunization up to date
　　　　Malaria pills (Chloroquine); also carry
　　　　Fansidar, unless sensitive to sulfa drugs

Malaria risk high; drug resistance widespread.
See "Malaria" in Sections II and III.

*high risk of diarrhea

II
INFORMATION ON
SPECIFIC IMMUNIZATIONS

If a "required" vaccine is not given on medical grounds, a statement to this effect should be made in the international certificate, signed by a physician, and validated.

Persons with immune-deficiencies (AIDS, those undergoing chemotherapy) should not receive live vaccines (such as yellow fever). They may receive killed vaccines (such as cholera, polio/Salk, tetanus, typhoid).

1
CHOLERA

Cholera immunizations are not generally necessary to protect travelers. They are recommended to facilitate entry into countries that request them for travelers arriving from areas that might have reported cholera cases.

IMMUNIZATION

One injection of 0.5 ml is sufficient for validation of the International Certificate and, for practical purposes, enough for travel.

TIMING

If two injections are given (only for special high risk areas), one to five weeks apart.

This is not a live vaccine; it may be given at the same time as other immunizations, or at any other time.

VALIDITY

From the sixth day after the first injection, for six months. The yellow Certificate must be validated by a health authority.

EFFECTIVENESS

Only moderate. Food and drink precautions still apply.

CHILDREN

Require proportionately smaller doses; infants under the age of one year are exempt.

REACTIONS

Local discomfort, sometimes fever and general malaise for a day or two. If reactions are more severe, do not give second injection.

BOOSTER

After six months, a 0.4-ml injection for prolonged or repeated trips. No matter how long ago the first immunization was given, only one booster injection is needed.

2
DIPHTHERIA, COMMUNICABLE CHILDHOOD DISEASES

Traveling children should be adequately immunized against them.

3
HEPATITIS—
IMMUNE (GAMMA) GLOBULIN

IMMUNIZATION

One 2-ml injection of immune globulin (gamma globulin) is suffficient for an adult of average weight for periods of up to two months. If exposure to the disease will be longer than two months, 1 ml per month is added to the 2-ml injection, up to a maximum of 5 ml for a six-month period. A dose of 5 ml should be repeated semiannually if exposure continues.

TIMING

As close as possible to departure time, since the effectiveness decreases with time.

Immune globulin does not affect yellow fever or polio immunizations, or killed vaccines (such as cholera, plague, tetanus, typhoid). It can be given at the same time as these, or at any other convenient time. Immune globulin may interfere with the response to some live vaccines (such as measles, mumps, rubella). Time permitting, intervals of four to twelve weeks are preferred.

CHILDREN

Proportionately smaller doses are required; none for infants.

REACTION

Generally none.

INDICATIONS

For travelers visiting only cities or resorts and using reasonable caution in the selection of food and eating places, the routine use of immune globulin is not essential. It may be warranted, however, for those visitors who do not limit their travel to ordinary tourist routes. Transmission of hepatitis usually takes place through uncooked foods or contaminated water and beverages.

4
JAPANESE ENCEPHALITIS

Immunization not recommended for travelers on tourist routes or for short term visitors.

Vaccination should be considered only for travelers who plan long term residence in farming areas of Southeast Asia and Japan.

Risk: remote.

Vaccine may be obtained through CDC (303-221-6429).

5
MALARIA

See also Section III, No. 14 on this topic.

PROPHYLAXIS

Malaria is a serious and growing health hazard to travelers. Chloroquine phosphate (Aralen) still provides reasonably good protection in many malarious areas. However, drug resistance is a growing problem.

IMMUNIZATION AND TIMING

One 500-mg tablet of chloroquine phosphate once a week, beginning a week before reaching a malarious region, continuing through the visit, and for six weeks after. If prophylaxis is impossible prior to arrival, two tablets may be taken on the first day.

Episodes of intestinal infection with diarrhea and vomiting may interfere with the absorption of chloroquine. In such cases, it is advisable to swallow an extra pill to maintain an adequate blood level of the drug.

PREGNANCY

Chloroquine may be taken during pregnancy.

CHILDREN

Require proportionately smaller amounts. Chloroquine phosphate is available in 500 mg and in 250-mg scored tablets.

For children, the taste of chloroquine may be disguised with sugar or chocolate syrup. Caution is advised, however, since excessive doses of chloroquine are toxic.

CHLOROQUINE-RESISTANT STRAINS

Occur in regions of South America, Africa, Southeast Asia, and the Western Pacific. Chloroquine will usually suffice for short visits to these areas when precautions such as screening, repellents, and long sleeves can be used during evening and night hours.

If exposure to chloroquine-resistant strains is likely, a physician should prescribe for each traveler one treatment dose (three tablets) of Fansidar (Roche), which combines 500 mg sulfadoxine with 25 mg pyrimethamine. Because of the occasional occurrence of severe toxic reactions to this drug, its routine use is discouraged unless the risk of exposure to drug-resistance malaria is high.

If a traveler to a region with drug-resistant organisms develops flu-like symptoms, chills, and fever, signs suggestive of malaria, medical care should be sought promptly. If this is not possible, three tablets of Fansidar should be taken, once, provided there is no known sensitivity to sulfa drugs. Children receive proportionately smaller doses.

Medical care should still be sought as quickly as feasible. Weekly doses of chloroquine should be continued.

If chloroquine is poorly tolerated, travelers may take Plaquenil (Winthrop), two 200-mg tablets a week, or one 200-mg tablet twice a week, with meals.

ALTERNATE PREVENTIVE TREATMENT OF MALARIA (for short term visitors)

Doxycycline, 100 mg daily (without taking chloroquine or Fansidar), while in the malarial area and for 10 days after. Children 8 to 11: 50 mg per day, depending on weight.

Doxycycline should not be taken during pregnancy and by children under age 8.
Caution: It may produce photosensitivity, with increased tendency to sunburn.
Despite all precautions, it is still possible to acquire malaria.

6
MENINGOCOCCAL DISEASE

Immunization for travelers not generally recommended. A vaccine is available (Menomune, Squibb-Connaught) for those who plan prolonged, close contact with local populations in Nepal. (Remote risk also in New Delhi.)

7
PLAGUE

IMMUNIZATION

Three injections of 0.5, 0.5, and 0.2 ml, in that order. No certification is required.

TIMING

Four weeks apart if time permits, or three weeks apart. This is not a live vaccine. It may be given at the same time as other immunizations, or at any other time.

EFFECTIVENESS

One year.

CHILDREN

Require proportionately smaller doses; no age limit.

REACTIONS

Some local pain, mild fever, and malaise.

BOOSTER

A single 0.2-ml injection after a year. The full course need never be repeated.

Immunization against plague is unnecessary for most travelers. Exceptions: persons going to Vietnam, Cambodia, Laos, and those who may be occupationally exposed to wild rodents.

8
POLIO

If the itinierary includes countries of low sanitary standards, children and young adults should receive a booster dose of oral vaccine that combines all polio strains.

This is a live virus vaccine. Other live virus vaccines (such as yellow fever) may be given on the same day or in any convenient time interval.

For adults older than 19, the injectable killed polio vaccine (Salk vaccine) is preferable. It is manufactured by Connaught Laboratories and is available in the United States.

9
RABIES

Pre-exposure immunization is recommended only for travelers who, through their high risk occupations, are likely to be exposed to animals in areas where rabies is prevalent.

IMMUNIZATION

Three intramuscular injections of 1 ml each, or equally effective, three intradermal injections of 0.1 ml each.

Imovax (Merieux) human diploid vaccine is available premeasured in syringes.

The intradermal injection should be given in the outer aspect of the upper arm.

TIMING

Second dose one week after first; third dose four weeks after first dose.

BOOSTER

0.1 ml intradermally, after one to three years, depending on exposure to risk.

10
SMALLPOX

All countries have lifted the requirement for this inoculation, thanks to the success of the World Health Organization in eradicating smallpox.

11
TETANUS

A tetanus booster is effective for 10 years. If a traveler is uncertain when he had his last tetanus injection, he should receive a booster and have the date entered on the yellow Certificate's appropriate page for future reference. There are no legal requirements in this respect.

Booster doses of 0.2 or 0.3 ml are adequate. They are less likely to cause adverse effects than larger doses.

12
TYPHOID FEVER

IMMUNIZATION AND TIMING

Two 0.5-ml injections, a month apart, or three injections at weekly intervals, if time does not permit the other schedule. No certification is required.

This is not a live vaccine. It may be given at the same time as other vaccines or, preferably, at any other time.

EFFECTIVENESS

Three years.

CHILDREN

Require proportionately smaller doses, at same intervals, but none for infants younger than one year.

REACTIONS

Local soreness, malaise, and fever for one or two days. If

there was a considerable reaction to the first or to a previous typhoid injection, the booster dose should be reduced.

BOOSTER

A single 0.5-ml injection after three years is recommended, but no matter how much time has elapsed since the last immunization, a single booster injection is sufficient.

Paratyphoid A & B (PAB) were, in the past, combined with typhoid vaccine. Because the reactions are more severe and the effectiveness is considered doubtful, the combination is no longer recommended.

13
TYPHUS

The effectiveness of this vaccine is questionable and its use is no longer recommended.

14
YELLOW FEVER

IMMUNIZATION

One injection, obtainable in special vaccination centers.

TIMING

If yellow fever and other live virus inoculations are needed, they may be given at the same time or in any convenient time interval.

Immune globulin does not interfere with response to yellow fever immunization.

VALIDITY

Ten days after immunization, for ten years. The yellow Certificate must be validated by a health authority.

CHILDREN

Recommended for children one year and older. Children 6-12 months can be exempt "on medical grounds." A physician's statement to this effect should be entered and signed in the International Certificate, and validated.

PREGNANCY

Yellow fever vaccination is not recommended (statement by physician required).

REACTIONS

Usually none.

BOOSTER

After ten years.

III
FOREIGN TRAVEL
HEALTH GUIDE

1
FOOD

RECOMMENDED (in developing countries)
Meat, preferably well done
Fish, fried or well cooked
Boiled eggs
Vegetables, cooked and served hot
Bread and other dry, baked goods

PRECAUTION
Wash hands before eating.

AVOID (in developing countries)
Salads (rinsing ingredients will not make them safe)
Undercooked (rare) meat
Sausages
Raw fish and shellfish
Most desserts (pies, custards, gelatins, creamy desserts)

In areas of questionable sanitary standards, the following rules should be observed even in first-class restaurants and hotels. (While the front desk may be elegant, the quality of the food handling in the kitchen is an unknown factor.) True, the gourmet traveler looks forward to savoring exotic dishes in foreign lands. Such gastronomical adventures carry little risk if the food comes to the table piping hot and if a few simple rules are observed.

When visiting tropical and subtropical countries: Eat food that has been freshly cooked and is still hot when served. Accept fruit only with skin intact, so that you can peel and core it yourself. If taking a day trip, hard-boiled eggs are good, safe sustenance as long as you can break the shell yourself. In countries with questionable hygienic standards, avoid lettuce and other salad ingredients, and any dishes made with mayonnaise, dressings, custards, and cream fillings.

Insist on well-done meat, even if you usually prefer it rare or medium-rare. This ensures that trichinae, various tapeworms, and other pathogens are killed in the cooking process.

The same applies to fish and other seafood. Raw seafood can be dangerous even in highly developed areas such as the Mediterranean. Many cases of hepatitis have been acquired in well-known eating places along the Riviera. As a rule, since fish tends to spoil quickly, it is wise not to eat fish unless you're near the water it's likely to have come from. And fish and other seafood should be avoided altogether if they are available only raw or undercooked.

Hepatitis A is widely prevalent in South Asia and Africa, and prophylactic immune globulin is recommended for travel in such high-risk areas, even for those who intend to eat only in first-class hotels and restaurants.

There is a myth that hot (meaning spicy) cuisine decreases contamination levels. Though the food may seem to burn a hole in the palate, that is no protection against pathogens.

2
BEVERAGES AND WATER

RECOMMENDED (in developing countries)
Hot tea, coffee, or soup
Boiled water
Beer

Wine (in corked bottles)
Carbonated soft drinks, mineral water (in sealed bottles or
    cans)
Canned milk

AVOID
Ice (Do not make an exception for alcoholic drinks.)
Water from pitchers or carafes in hotel rooms
Fresh milk (unless boiled)
Milk products
Ice cream
Cheeses (except for known brands in original packaging)

Hot climates—and even mild bouts of diarrhea—can de-
plete body fluids and call for increased liquid intake.

Hot soups, consomme, tea, and coffee are safe. Iced tea or
coffee, though thirst-quenching, can be contaminated by
ice cubes made from impure water.

Fruit, if you can peel it yourself, safely provides needed
liquid, and oranges and grapefruit are particularly good
because they offer vitamin C along with their juice. (However, fruit should be avoided during and immediately
following diarrhea.)

In countries with poor sanitary standards, it's wiser to
avoid beverages of unknown brand. Fortunately, most
countries today have bottling plants that produce carbonated soft drinks under familiar brand labels, and these
franchised bottlers are usually inspected by parent-com-
pany representatives. Such products are generally safe to
consume if purchased with an unopened seal or cap.

Water from the hot tap, if it's hot enough to feel uncom-
fortable on the hand, is, for all practical purposes, pasteurized and, after cooling, safe enough for oral hygiene,
diluting drinks, or washing eating utensils. Cold tap

water, which some tourists unthinkingly use for tooth-brushing or to dilute drinks, can be a source of infection.

Another caveat: Don't drink bulk-stored water on trains, planes, or any public conveyance. Hot tea or coffee and bottled or canned drinks will quench thirst as well—and more safely.

Questionable drinking water may be treated by mixing it in a container with a chlorine or iodine preparation. Various purifying tablets (such as Halazone or Potable-Aqua) are available in army surplus stores, drugstores, etc. Follow the directions on the package.

Do not drink the untreated water in carafes or pitchers placed in your hotel room. It is usually more contaminated than the tap water.

On long plane rides, the body's water loss is considerable. To avoid dehydration, drink any of the beverages recommended above.

Giardiasis is an infection acquired from drinking water, and the causative parasite, *Giardia lamblia*, is found worldwide. While the disease occasionally seems to hit tourists coming home from the Soviet Union, it is not uncommon in other cool regions.

Usually, there is a delay in the onset of symptoms—well after journey's end, unlike the "trots," which will occur during or immediately after a trip. Giardiasis symptoms may include diarrhea, fatigue, weight loss, cramps, and nausea. In mild cases, the only complaints may be tiredness and inexplicable malaise. Good drugs are available to treat the infection, but diagnosis can be difficult.

There is no immunization against giardiasis, so to guard against it, do as the Russians do: Drink hot tea.

3
ICE AND ALCOHOLIC DRINKS

Ice can be a troublemaker for travelers abroad. It's prepared from unboiled water and often handled in a careless manner, as if freezing were bactericidal. It's not. So, unless you are sure of the hotel's or the country's health standards, order un-iced drinks. In fact, you should learn the key phrase, "without ice," in every language you are likely to encounter.

Some people believe that alcohol kills bacteria. Hard liquor, taken undiluted, is safe—bacteriologically, at least. If combined with bottled mixers of reputable brands, it will also be safe. But alcohol in punches, mixed cocktails, and so on, does *not* disinfect the mixture—at least, not rapidly or reliably.

Beer and wine are generally acceptable drinks if brought to the table in their original, unopened bottles. Otherwise, who can tell what's been added to the brew? In some countries, an occasional innkeeper will make a practice of adulterating the wine, and ordering a carafe may not be advisable.

4
MILK AND ICE CREAM

A strong word of caution: Except in countries that have high standards of hygiene, do not drink milk unless it has been heated to boiling point.

Canned evaporated or condensed milk is safe and available in most places. If you want to dilute it, add boiled water.

Beware of milk containers labeled "pasteurized." In some foreign countries, that's no guarantee that the proper heating process was used.

Ice cream and other milk/cream products are foods to avoid altogether in most tropical countries. This includes cheeses, unless they are known brands, still in their original packaging.

5
VITAMINS

The traveler who limits his diet to avoid intestinal infections may feel that vitamin supplementation is required. It will do no harm but is hardly necessary if the trip is to last only a few weeks.

Vitamin A and D deficiencies won't develop in such a short period of time. Vitamin C is found in oranges, grapefruit, or other peelable fruit—but don't rely on bananas as a C source. The B complex vitamins are contained in the average tourist menu: meat, vegetables, cereal, eggs, and so on.

If a prolonged stay is contemplated in areas where strict dietary precautions are recommended, a daily, simple vitamin supplement (not a therapeutic formula) may be used.

Children, particularly infants, should continue their regular, prescribed vitamin combinations while traveling.

6
DIARRHEA: PREVENTION/TREATMENT

What makes a tourist run? Diarrhea—known as Delhi Belly in India, Montezuma's Revenge in Mexico, Mummy Tummy in Egypt, and elsewhere as the trots, the GIs, or La Turista.

It is caused by a great variety of microorganisms, in addition to dysentery producers such as *Shigella*, *Salmonella*, and amebae. Also responsible are many bacilli common everywhere but which, in hot climates, can proliferate and produce severe symptoms when ingested.

High-risk destinations include most of the developing countries of Latin America, Africa, the Middle East, and Asia. Most of the southern European countries and some of the Caribbean islands are regions of moderate risk. Low-risk destinations include Canada, most of Europe, Australia, and New Zealand.

The more protected a traveler's home environment, the more he'll be affected in areas of poor sanitation; and the tourist from a temperate zone will tend to suffer more than one arriving from the tropics or subtropics.

Will frequent trips and gradual exposure to alien microorganisms and bacilli build up a traveler's immunity? Not really. Even the natives of warm countries with low sanitary standards are afflicted by diarrhea, sometimes severely. The safest road to follow is careful selection of food and drink. (Check the chapters on those subjects.)

But if you do develop diarrhea, despite all precautions, what can be done?

In an emergency situation—blood in the stools, consider-able dehydration, vomiting, or fever—a physician is needed. Otherwise, the following advice is offered:

Do not force yourself to eat if you have no appetite. Drink lots of liquids, such as weak tea or boiled water. Sugar, honey, or syrup may be added, but no milk. A few drops of lemon for flavoring is also permissible.

Take soups, bouillon, or consomme served hot. They're good because they contain salt, which has been depleted in the body during the ailment's acute phase. (Bouillon cubes are easy to carry, easy to prepare.)

Cola drinks and other carbonated beverages of known brands are permissible but avoid fruit and vegetables for at least three days. Orange juice or well-chewed bananas are permissible, even beneficial, since they contain potassium.

Use a hot water bottle to help alleviate stomach cramps.

When the appetite returns, eat lightly for a few days. Start with boiled rice, cooked cereals, poached or boiled eggs, and the old standby—hot soup. Later, add lean, well-done meats and bananas (no other fruit) to the diet. When all symptoms have vanished, eat—but selectively!

7
DIARRHEA:
MEDICATION

It is not advisable to take medication to prevent diarrhea.

However, when traveling in developing countries you should take along medication that slows down an overactive bowel, such as Imodium (loperamide) or a bottle of paregoric. In acute diarrhea, the dosage of Imodium is 2 capsules (4 mg), followed by 1 capsule after each diarrheal stool, up to 8 capsules a day. Paregoric: 1 teaspoon, up to 4 times a day.

An alternative is Pepto Bismol (bismuth subsalicylate) 1 oz every 30 minutes.

It is not advisable to exceed the dosage recommended on the package or by a physician, to take such drugs for more than two days, or to give them to small children.

Should diarrhea continue and local medical help be unavailable, then doxycycline with its fairly broad range of effectiveness may be tried. The suggested regimen is one 100-mg tablet or capsule a day for several days.

Occasionally, such a short course of an antibiotic may be indicated. But since a variety of bacteria, viruses, or other organisms may be involved, the response to any one antibiotic cannot be predicted.

Bactrim or Septra (trimethoprim-sulfamethoxazol) should not be taken, unless advised by a physician.

When there is fever, blood in the stool, vomiting, or signs of dehydration, medical care is a matter of urgency, even if it means traveling further to reach properly equipped facilities.

Various antidiarrheals with unfamiliar names can be bought without prescription in some countries, but let the traveler beware! In particular, avoid chloromycetin and Entero-Vioform, which are still popular in many developing countries. They are potentially toxic.

8
CONSTIPATION

Though less worrisome or dramatic than diarrhea, constipation affects some travelers, especially those visiting cooler climates. The intestines tend to become sluggish because daily routine has been disturbed. Unattractive, unfamiliar toilets are additional inhibiting factors. But some simple steps can help prevent constipation.

Don't postpone taking care of physical needs before leaving home or boarding planes. The small, cramped toilets on planes are not conducive to relaxed, satisfying emptying of the bowels.

Drink plenty of liquids while traveling, even more than thirst demands. Eat fresh fruit—the safe, peel-it-yourself variety.

If the problem persists, or if you normally tend to be constipated, a mild laxative will give relief. Milk of magnesia can be taken along or purchased in drugstores just about everywhere. Pharmacists abroad may also suggest Epsom salts, but they can keep a tourist hotel-bound for precious hours or days.

Diarrhea is frequently followed by constipation. That's merely the body's way of allowing the intestines to regain their normal rhythm, and medication is contraindicated.

9
TRAVELING WITH
A COLD

Common dilemma: A cold and departure time for a long-anticipated trip arrive simultaneously. Upper respiratory infections are special problems for air travelers, who generally can not—or will not—rearrange their flight schedules.

Air pressure in modern jet planes corresponds to altitudes of 5,000-8,000 feet above sea level, leaving plenty of oxygen for the resting, healthy passenger. But for the traveler with a cold, this pressure may result in a bulging and painful eardrum.

To minimize cold discomfort and earache, the adult traveler should use a nasal decongestant before boarding the plane, and a nasal spray during ascent and descent. (It is advisable to start approximately a half hour before the scheduled descent.) Chewing gum or, even better, small sips taken frequently from a bottle of liquid held for this purpose, can prove very helpful. Taking such sips at take-off, before landing, and during periods of changing altitudes, helps to restore equalized pressure in the head's air spaces, and to reduce ear pain, which can be severe when the eustachian tubes are clogged. Yawning is helpful, too.

It's worth remembering that the flight crew is not permitted to serve beverages (not even water) while the plane is ascending or descending. In any case, small sips of your own liquid supply will do a better job than the candies dispensed by some airlines.

Should swallowing or yawning fail to help, a technique that often provides relief during descent is this: try forcing air out through the nose, mouth closed, while holding both nostrils closed with thumb and index finger. In so doing, you will gradually increase the pressure, opening the eustachian tubes. If successful, there will be a popping sound, and with it the pain will be relieved. This maneuver may have to be repeated several times. This will *not* work when the plane is climbing. However, descent causes greater discomfort than ascent.

Best of all, avoid flying with a head cold, if possible.

10
THE TRAVELER
WITH HEALTH PROBLEMS

RECOMMENDED
A physician's letter describing the condition and medication being taken
A "dog tag" indicating major problems or allergies
Medications, carried in original, labeled containers

DIABETES
Diabetics should increase insulin dose by 25 per cent for six time zones, flying west; and decrease it by 25 per cent for six time zones, flying east (to compensate for longer or shorter days).

CARDIAC CONDITIONS
Some people with limited cardiac or pulmonary reserve may experience difficulties at altitudes over 6,000 feet. The atmosphere in the pressurized cabin of a jet plane corresponds to 5,000-8,000 feet.

Federal regulations do not permit a personal oxygen container to be taken aboard a plane. Exceptions cannot be made, even with letters from physicians. However, every jet plane carries oxygen for first-aid purposes. If a larger supply may be needed, the airline should be notified in advance—and a small tank will be installed under the seat. The airlines do not charge for emergency oxygen, but do charge for providing such a tank.

With such standby provisions, and with the permission of his physician, a cardiac patient may be able to travel four weeks after suffering a heart attack.

11
HANDICAPPED
AND AGED TRAVELERS

The Federal Aviation Administration (FAA) has published a guidebook that helps make travel easier for the handicapped and the aged. "Access Travel: Airports" describes the facilities and services available to meet the needs of travelers requiring wheelchairs, as well as those who are blind and deaf. It includes information about 282 airport terminals in 40 countries.

The pamphlet lists such features as special ramps, reserved parking, accessible restrooms, telephones with amplifiers, and special transportation. Single, free copies can be obtained by writing to the Architectural and Transportation Barriers Compliance Board, Washington, D.C. 20202.

12
OTHER ILLNESSES

Travelers with chronic or temporary medical disorders must take along their medication, of course, but in original, proper pharmacy containers. That will prevent unpleasant drug-regulation incidents at airports or country borders. In addition, carrying extra supplies is a good idea, because many of the drugs used at home are unobtainable abroad or available only by different names and in different concentrations.

The ailing individual staying abroad for longer than a usual vacation period should ask his physician for type-written prescriptions stating both trade and generic names of the drugs, and dosage given in the metric system.

The unlucky traveler who gets sick en route should not consult pharmacists or even physicians, unless they've been recommended by reputable sources. (See Section III, No. 17.)

Eyeglass wearers: Carry a prescription in case replacements are needed. They can be purchased with little trouble, at relatively low cost, in most countries.

Diabetics on insulin may need to modify their dosages, as mentioned in Section III, No. 10. Going east, the journey day may be five, six, or more hours shorter than the ordinary 24 hours; accordingly, insulin dosage is cut by 15 to 25 per cent. The opposite is true going west, when days stretch correspondingly. Diabetics should discuss this with their physicians before departing.

Similar modifications may apply to other medications, although few have dosages so exactly calculated as insulin. A small difference during one day in most drug regimens is relatively unimportant.

How do some travelers come by the exotic diseases caused by microorganisms or parasites not found at home? Primarily through food, drink, and insect bites—only rarely by direct contact with infected objects.

A noteworthy exception to this are Haitian handicrafts made from goatskin.

RECOMMENDED

TO PREVENT AIDS: In countries with low sanitary standards, avoid blood transfusions, if at all possible. Also keep away from tattoos and avoid local sexual contacts.

When in Haiti, do not buy products made from goatskin. Many such skins are contaminated with the anthrax bacillus, which can produce serious infections.

13
ACCIDENTS AND INJURIES

When an accident or injury requires medical treatment, the attending physician should be told if the traveler has had a recent tetanus toxoid booster. Another small booster may be deemed necessary, but a tetanus antiserum injection—with possibly unpleasant consequences—may be avoided.

Circumstances permitting, travelers should consult surgeons or physicians recommended by consulates or university hospitals.

Minor injuries are almost inevitable in strange surroundings. Abrasions or cuts can be expected from sharp-edged furniture, a piece of metal or glass on a beach, can openers, the doors of a rickety cab, and so on. The rule is to wash the injury with soap and water as soon as feasible, and cover it with a Band-Aid adhesive bandage or similar dressing. Don't use iodine, Mercurochrome, or any other antiseptic.

14
MALARIA

Malaria, still the most widespread of all human diseases, is prevalent in large parts of Central and South America, Africa, and Asia. Prevention is important. (For details, see Section II, No. 5.)

Many travelers are unaware of the danger of malaria or choose to ignore it. This can prove foolhardy. Keep in mind that mosquitoes strike most frequently between dusk and dawn, so special precautions should be taken during this period.

RECOMMENDED (after sunset)
Stay in areas that are screened in.

Wear light-colored clothing (dark colors attract mosquitoes more than light colors)
Apply mosquito-repellent lotions or sprays (containing DEET) to exposed skin
Wear long sleeves and pants
Take preventive medication regularly
Avoid perfume, toilet water, and scented soaps
Avoid after-shave lotion

Nowhere is malaria prophylaxis a legal requirement. Responsibility for precautionary measures lies with the traveler. In some countries listed as malarious, the disease is confined to limited, rural areas, and visiting major cities is less hazardous. However, omitting the medication may prevent you from taking side trips or changing plans.

If exposure to malaria is unlikely (because the visit will be short or the disease is not common in the region) other preventive measures may be adequate. Insect-repellent sprays, lotions, and sticks do protect—but only if applied *before* the mosquito bites. Unfortunately, tourists often wait until they're reminded by the first sting. That can happen at any time of day or night, though the anopheles mosquito favors 5 P.M. through 7 A.M. for feasting on humans.

In infested regions, other worthwhile protection comes from mosquito nets, window screens, and long pants and sleeves worn after dusk, in addition to repellents applied to exposed body parts.

While taking any medication during pregnancy is undesirable, malaria presents a greater risk. The World Health Organization considers antimalarial medication to be safe for mothers-to-be who are traveling. (The sulfadoxine-pyrimethamine combination, however, is not recommended for pregnant women or nursing mothers. See Section II. No. 5.)

The 500-mg chloroquine tablet (the adult dose for malaria prevention) is coated. In the U.S., the drug is not available in a pediatric suspension. 250-mg scored tablets, however, are available. One such tablet may be given to children weighing 60 to 110 pounds, half a tablet to those weighing 30 to 60 pounds, and a quarter tablet to those weighing less than that.

Chloroquine has a bitter taste. If used for children, the tablet should be crushed and the taste disguised by mixing it with a quarter teaspoon of sugar, or with chocolate syrup.

15
HOW TO GET HOME IF ILL OR INJURED ABROAD

Assistance in obtaining emergency transportation can usually be obtained through the nearest American or Canadian consul.

In many areas, private air ambulances are available but they are extremely expensive, and sometimes payment in advance is required. However, such ambulances may often be the preferred method for local transport or to connect with a major airline equipped to transport the ill or injured. In some parts of the world, U.S. military evacuation can be obtained but this, too, can be quite costly.

U.S. carriers that transport the ill or injured do so according to special guidelines. If a sitting position is not possible, patients can be accommodated on stretchers, which many airlines provide. If feasible, arrangements should be made several days before flight time, through the airline reservation office. The airlines usually charge for four seats—for the stretcher and two accompanying passengers.

Some insurance companies offer policies that cover the expenses of getting home in case of a medical emergency. Nationwide Emergency Ambulance Return (NEAR), in

Oklahoma City, Okla. (800-654-6700), offers a service that will arrange for transportation home for ill or injured travelers who have paid an annual fee. This program is highly recommended, particularly for the older traveler.

16
PAIN KILLERS
AND TRANQUILIZERS

Codeine can come in handy, and travelers can take along a dozen or so 30-mg tablets (this requires a prescription). One tablet may be taken every four to six hours for major, debilitating conditions—bad colds, painful joints or muscles, or severe diarrhea, for example. Codeine, however, merely relieves the problem; it doesn't solve it.

Aspirin is available in pharmacies everywhere. It can be combined with codeine, if necessary.
People on sedatives at home will likely continue their use while away. But for help in adapting to different time zones, even people who do not ordinarily take tranquilizers may find sedatives such as diazepam (Valium) or sleeping pills useful. See Section III. No. 23 on jet lag.

17
HOW TO FIND
A DOCTOR ABROAD

When a physician referral is needed, travelers can turn to U.S., Canadian, or British consulates; the nearest medical school or university hospital; and, naturally, to resident friends. American Express offices can sometimes help, too. When these means are not possible, a hotel manager may be able to recommend a physician. Generally speaking, it's better not to ask the local pharmacists for their recommendations.

Being prepared is, of course, the best method of locating doctors abroad. Several responsible associations supply such information. Lists from IAMAT, the International Association for Medical Assistance to Travelers, 417 Center Street, Lewiston, NY 14092, are highly recommended. See Section III, No. 31 for a partial list of IAMAT centers.

If all else fails, you can try to reach IAMAT's Toronto office by overseas phone and request the name of a recommended, English-speaking physician. The phone number is: Canada's country code plus 519-836-0102. The call should, of course, be placed during Toronto office hours.

Anyone incurring medical or hospital expenses while abroad should ask for receipted bills. They may be covered by American medical insurance companies and the Blue Cross/Blue Shield plans, but not by Medicare.

In most hotels in the world, "I need a doctor" will probably be understood when said in English. If not, one of these languages will almost certainly be understood:

German: Ich brauche einen Arzt.

French: J'ai besoin d'un médecin.

Spanish: Deseo ver un medico.

Italian: Desidero vedere un medico.

Portuguese: Desejo ver um médico.

18
PLANE TRAVEL

RECOMMENDED (for long plane trips)

Take daylight rather than night flights whenever possible

Select seats close to the front of the plane

Request an aisle seat rather than a window seat

Get up and stretch your limbs once in a while, or take short strolls in the aisle

Wear loose clothing, or loosen it while in your seat

Put on slippers carried aboard in hand luggage

Drink more than usual, but very little alcohol (wine is preferable to hard liquor)

Eat moderately

Avoid smoking

Avoid flying with a head cold (see Section III, No. 9)

Use the toilet before boarding the plane

Pack the minimum compatible with trip comfort (on arrival, porters are often unavailable and you may have to carry your luggage)

Going north, east, south, or west, daylight flights are always less tiring. Some people are able to sleep fairly well on planes, but even so, this affords only a partial rest and leaves much to be desired. If night flights are necessary, earplugs and eyeshades, which can be purchased at most airports, are helpful in getting rest. In general, try to get a seat as far forward as your plane ticket permits, since the back of the plane tends to be noisier.

The atmosphere on a jet plane is drier than desert air. For this reason, it is advisable to drink more fluids than usual. Alcohol, however, has a much stronger effect at high altitudes and should be consumed in small quantities, if at all, while airborne.

On longer flights, it's a good idea to leave your seat and move around once in a while, stretching your muscles. This is not only beneficial to the joints and the blood circulation, but also makes you feel more comfortable when you return to your seat.

19
HEALTH PROBLEMS AT HIGH ALTITUDES

RECOMMENDED

If possible, allow for a day or two of intermediate stops before ascending to altitudes higher than 8,000 feet (2,500 meters)

Limit exertion for first few days, till adaptation is achieved

If trouble arises, inhale oxygen; return to lower altitudes

Do not use sleeping pills or sedatives, since they reduce breathing and, therefore, oxygen intake

Acclimatization takes about two days for healthy individuals at altitudes of 8-9,000 feet, longer for higher altitudes. Symptoms may include headache, loss of appetite, nausea, palpitations, and fatigue. These usually disappear in a few days, as acclimatization occurs.

Occasionally, travelers experience swelling of face, hands, or feet. This may last for days, or even longer.

A more serious illness, seen occasionally after heavy exertion at higher altitudes, causes "waterlogged" lungs (lung edema). It occurs in young people—even children—as much as in older people. Shortness of breath and coughing are the first signs. Oxygen and prompt return to lower altitudes are necessary in such cases.

20
TRAVEL IN CHINA

Since the People's Republic of China opened its borders to visitors in 1976, the number of people traveling there has jumped by leaps and bounds, and some health recommendations seem to be in order.

Travelers to China frequently develop upper respiratory infections during their stay. Gastrointestinal problems, ranging from mild to disabling, are also common. Since it is not possible to find familiar remedies, it is best to come prepared with what you might need.

Two factors encourage the spread of infection. First, much of the tourist transportation within the country is by bus. Sitting for many hours in a closed environment near someone with an upper respiratory infection certainly increases the chances of acquiring it.

Second, the meals, often consisting of 10 or 12 different dishes, are served family style. But serving spoons are rare. Diners use their individual chopsticks to shovel food off the platters and onto their plates; some also use them to stir the sauce on the platters. If one member of the group has a communicable ailment (a sore throat, for instance), his chopsticks, with which he has just eaten his previous course, can infect the food on the next platter that is passed.

RECOMMENDED
With the help of your group interpreter, ask the waiter for a serving spoon. Or carry a card with the request written in Chinese characters, and show it to the waiter when the first platter is brought out.

Many of the dishes offered are unfamiliar to Americans. Travelers to China tend to overeat when so many delicacies are placed before them. Flatulence, diarrhea, or constipation often result.

RECOMMENDED
Take along some charcoal capsules, an over-the-counter medication that helps absorb intestinal gas. And see the chapters on diarrhea and constipation (Section III, Nos. 6, 7, and 8) for additional remedies. But don't take a laxative in the evening if your next sightseeing tour or bus trip begins at 5 or 6 A.M. (not unusual in China). The medication may decide to act when you're nowhere near a bathroom.

Water placed in your room in a pitcher is supposedly boiled. But don't count on it. See Section III, No. 2 for advice on brushing teeth and other uses of water.

The temperatures in the Beijing (Peking) area are likely to be approximately what they would be, at the same time of year, in southern New England. Should inclement weather strike unexpectedly, you may not be able to warm up indoors. Many of the hotels and guest houses do not have heat till midwinter, if at all, and the buildings have a way of retaining frigid and clammy air.

RECOMMENDED
If you plan to be in northern China (and visit the Great Wall) between September and May, take along a warm coat and sweater, some lightweight ski underwear (which you can sleep in if necessary), gloves, and heavy socks— all of which may become especially useful at night.

If your trip is in the spring or fall, be sure to take along a folding umbrella. The sightseeing goes on, no matter how heavy the rain.

21
PREGNANCY AND TRAVEL

Officially, the airlines will accept a pregnant traveler through the eighth month of pregnancy. After that, they are acting within regulations if they require a note from her physician clearing her for the flight.

Pleasure trips to countries with low sanitary standards are not recommended during the first few months of pregnancy. However, if travel is inescapable, pregnant women should avoid medication of any sort, pre-trip immunizations included. Especially hazardous are the attenuated viral materials used in yellow fever, polio, measles, and German measles inoculations. While typhoid and cholera immunizations are relatively safe, they too are better avoided during the first trimester.

One exception: malaria prophylaxis. The disease has greater risks than those of antimalarial medication. Fansidar (the sulfadoxine-pyrimethamine combination) is not recommended for pregnant women or nursing mothers. See Section II, No. 5, and Section III, No. 14.

22
TRAVEL WITH CHILDREN

Children have a greater tendency to motion sickness than adults. If such a tendency is evident, the child should be seated as far forward as possible if traveling by bus; on the front rather than the back seat in a car.

During air travel, children suffer more readily from earaches during the ascent, and even more so during the descent. The ducts linking the middle ear with the nasal cavity are narrower in children, making it more difficult for air pressure in the ear and nose to equalize when the pressure in the plane changes.

RECOMMENDED
Bottle-feed an infant during a plane's descent. If the infant is not hungry, give a bottle of water. The frequent swallowing helps equalize the air pressure in the ear and nose. If traveling with small children, give them something to induce swallowing—a liquid, chewing gum, or candy. Lemon or lime flavors are preferable because they stimulate salivary flow. Since airline regulations prohibit the crew from serving during take-off and landing, those traveling with infants or children should carry such beverages or candy with them.

23
JET LAG

While jet lag occurs when flying in either direction, the experience of most people is that adaptation is easier when flying westward. A longer day appears to be more acceptable to the body and mind than a shorter one. In trips around the world, if you have a choice, go west. It will be less disturbing to the biological clock. To reduce jet lag on flights from west to east, morning or daylight flights are always preferable to night flights.

The most common symptoms of jet lag are tiredness, listlessness, irritability, and a slight headache. On arrival in daytime after long eastbound flights, it is advisable to wear sunglasses, to keep exertion to a minimum, and to catch a nap at the first possible opportunity.

We are ordinarily geared to function according to a 24-hour cycle. It's called the circadian rhythm, a word from the Latin "circa," *about*, and "diem," *day*.

Our habits and normal functioning of circulatory, digestive, and nervous systems have orderly highs and lows within each 24 hours. Disrupting the cycle by adding to or subtracting from the day plays havoc with organ functions and, occasionally, with intellectual capacity. The first few days' enjoyment is often diminished, and we remember places seen then as less attractive, and minor incidents as especially irritating. This applies less to daytime travel westward, since a good night's sleep after arrival is possible.

But everybody—except, perhaps, youngsters and unrushed tourists—suffers somewhat from jet lag. The average traveler needs about one day to adapt for every two hours of time change. Thus, jet lag is a big problem for people on short business trips, when physical endurance and quick decisions count heavily, and for tourists with sightseeing schedules that allow no time for rest-and-recovery periods.

Those traveling for important business should realize that for the first few days after eastbound flights, the best time for negotiations or decision-making is during afternoon hours; after westbound flights, the morning hours.

When the differential exceeds seven hours, a break in the trip (if possible, a layover for a day or two) promotes body readjustment. You might also do the following:

Go to bed the first night at the *local* bedtime, and take an "average dose" of an anti-insomnia drug—100 mg of secobarbital (Seconal) or 15 mg of flurazepam (Dalmane), for example, either of which must be purchased with prescription before departure. Go to bed the second night, again at local bedtime, and take a smaller dose of medication—i.e., open the capsule and discard part of its contents. By the third night, adaptation will have been accomplished in most cases.

Other helpful agents are 15-mg Serax or 2-mg diazepam (Valium) tablets. Both are procure-in-advance prescription drugs. Two tablets may be taken the first night; one tablet the second night; and one the third night if still needed.

It is best to avoid stimulants such as tea and coffee near the new bedtime, and wiser to take moderate-sized, non-adventurous meals for the first few days.

24
MOTION SICKNESS

Here's the curse of many a sea voyager. It affects air travelers, as well, although the speed of today's jet planes minimizes the risk, even for people who are prone to motion sickness.

The following helpful hints apply to sailors:

Recline as far as possible, or lie flat on your back, circumstances permitting. Do not read or watch movies. Remember that fresh air on the deck is better than cabin confinement. When the urge to vomit comes, don't hold back; it will relieve the symptoms, at least temporarily. Thereafter, eat something light and appealing to your palate: You may have to taste it again.

Medications taken to prevent motion sickness on plane or ship must be ingested early, or they won't be retained either. The popular agents are Dramamine and Bonine, and both are reasonably effective. But antihistamines are, too. So the traveler who anticipates motion sickness should carry appropriate drugs, some of which may be obtained without prescription.

25
TROPICAL HEAT

RECOMMENDED
Greatly increase non-alcoholic fluid intake
Decrease alcoholic intake
Add salt to food
Defer strenuous activities (jogging, tennis) until the cooler part of the day
Wear clothing and stockings or socks made of cotton
Avoid clothing made of synthetic materials (they do not absorb moisture and ventilate poorly; even nylon pantyhose are not recommended)
Wear white or light-colored fabrics (they are cooler than dark materials)
Wear a light hat with a brim
Use moderation in exposure to the sun, particularly during the first few days
Use sunscreen preparations
Avoid sneakers and footwear with rubber soles (they tend to retain moisture and encourage fungal growth)

Most people have little difficulty adapting to hot climates. Children and young persons are less affected by heat than older persons. However, since their skin tends to be moister, young people suffer more frequently from skin disorders, such as fungal infections. This is aggravated by the fact that younger people are partial to sneakers and other rubber-soled footwear, which promote the tendency to fungal infections (athlete's foot).

Some people experience moderate swelling of the ankles when visiting the tropics. In an otherwise healthy person, this can be disregarded as it is usually self-limiting. It is helpful to sit with the legs elevated and to avoid all tight clothing, including tight belts, knee socks with elasticized tops, and any garment that is held up with elastic around the waist or stomach.

26
GUARDING AGAINST INSECTS

Various infections, in addition to malaria, can be transmitted by insect stings. Precautions are important, especially in the tropics.

Repellents sprayed or applied to skin and clothing will keep insects away. Repellents are harmless to humans— provided the hands are washed before eating.

However, a distinction should be made between harmless insect repellents and the more toxic insecticides. The repellents can be used on the skin and clothing. But if a room has been sprayed with an insecticide, it is advisable to stay out of it for at least half an hour after the spraying.

Wearing long sleeves and long pants after dusk also cuts down insect targets.

When a traveler in an insect-infested region spends the night in an unscreened room—or hut or tent—he needs a sleeping net (nylon is better than cotton) and generous applications of insect repellents.

Ticks present another problem. They should be removed with tweezers, with a minimum of squeezing. A drop of gasoline, alcohol, or tincture of iodine applied first will help prevent breaking off the tick's head.

27
EARPLUGS
AND
EYECOVERS

Some travelers find it hard to sleep in strange, metropolitan hotels, selected because of good location—everything within walking distance. But it naturally follows that typical city noises will surround them.

To filter out some of the din, try earplugs. Though they take some getting used to, they can promote a good night's rest, especially for the chronically poor sleeper. And if the hotel should go up in flames, the earplug wearer can still hear the fire alarm.

Another trick is to request an inside room, away from city streets. What's sacrificed in views is compensated for in nightly peace.

Eyecovers are useful on planes and in east-facing hotel rooms invaded by light at 5 in the morning.

Both items are usually sold in drugstores and international airport shops.

28
FOOT CARE

Comfortable shoes are a most important travel accessory. If new shoes are part of the wardrobe, they should be broken in before departure.

On a long plane flight, wear light slippers (previously packed in the hand luggage) instead of shoes.

Feet tend to expand in warm or tropical climates, so check shoe size for extra room well in advance. Aching, cramped feet have spoiled many a vacation.

Fungal infections of the foot, common in warm climates, are usually slow in developing, and may not blossom during a short trip.

Proper sock fit is important, too. For comfort in hot climates, choose cotton socks. They absorb perspiration; nylon or other synthetics do not.

29
SWIMMING IN
STRANGE PLACES

NOT RECOMMENDED (in areas with poor sanitation and in some tropical regions)
Swimming, even wading, in fresh water in the regions mentioned below
Swimming off ocean beaches in the vicinity of cities (at least, keep your head out of the water)

RECOMMENDED
Swimming off ocean beaches not close to cities
Swimming in chlorinated pools

A wormlike parasite, the fluke known as schistosoma, can cause schistosomiasis, one symptom of which is blood in the urine. The parasite lives in the fresh water of ponds, lakes, and rivers in many regions, but is never found in salt or brackish water, or in swimming pools.

Swimming is probably safe in well-maintained, man-made pools or in places that, according to good authority, are free of schistosoma. Quell the urge to bathe in the *fresh* waters of:

Africa, including North Africa and Madagascar, and particularly the Nile River Valley and the Congo River Basin;

South America's northeastern portion, particularly the Amazon regions, parts of Brazil and Venezuela, and also the Caribbean Islands;

East Asia, particularly China and the Philippines. Schistosoma has, however, been eradicated in Japan and on the Island of Luzon.

30
MEDICINE KIT FOR TRAVEL

The areas to be visited should determine the medicine kit's contents. For general purposes, however, the following items are recommended:

Chloroquine (Aralen) for malarious regions
Immodium tablets or liquid

Tetracycline capsules, 250 mg: or doxycycline (Vibramycin) capsules, 100 mg

A few tranquilizer tablets, such as Valium, 2 or 5 mg; or Serax, 15 mg

Aspirin or acetaminophen (Tylenol)

A thermometer

Band-Aid adhesive bandages, or gauze and tape

31
CENTERS FOR MEDICAL ASSISTANCE TO TRAVELERS

For the international traveler, IAMAT (International Association for Medical Assistance to Travelers) is an organization worth joining. It is especially recommended for older travelers and those with health problems. There is no set membership fee, but voluntary contributions are invited. IAMAT publishes lists of centers where travelers can get information on qualified English-speaking doctors.

Following are the phone numbers for IAMAT centers around the world. This list is accurate as this book goes to press. However, in some countries information changes frequently. For updated and more complete listings, write to IAMAT, 417 Center Street, Lewiston, NY 14092.

ALGERIA
Algiers
Institut Pasteur d'Algerie
 Tel. 65 88 60

ANGOLA
Luanda
IAMAT Coord., Teresa Cohen, MD
 Tel. 22 886

ARGENTINA
Buenos Aires
IAMAT Center
 Tel. 791 9956
Hospital Britanico
 Tel. 23 1081/9

ARUBA
Oranjestad
Oduber Hospital
Tel. 43 00

AUSTRIA
Innsbruck
IAMAT Center
Tel. (05222) 24 314
Vienna
IAMAT Center, Walter Doralt, MD
Tel. 482 721

BAHAMAS
Freeport
IAMAT Coord., Neil A. Sawyer, MB
Tel. 373 4689

BANGLADESH
Dacca
Holy Family Hospital
Tel. 400 011

BELGIUM
Brussels
IAMAT Center
Tel. 537 7323

BELIZE
Belize City
IAMAT Center
Tel. 45 261

BENIN
Cotonou
IMAT Coord., Bruno Monteiro, MD
Tel. 315 773

BOLIVIA
La Paz
IAMAT Center
Tel. 371 826

BOTSWANA
Gabarone
IAMAT Coord., A.E. Bhoola, M.B.
2 610

BRAZIL
Brasilia
Casa de Saude Santa Lucia
Tel. 245 3344
Rio De Janeiro—Ipanema
IAMAT Coord., Roberto German, MD
Tel. 205 1491
Sao Paulo
IAMAT Center
Tel. 247 4918

BURUNDI
Bujumbura
IAMAT Center
Tel. 57 50

CAMEROON
Yaounde
IAMAT Center
Tel. 224 523

CANARY ISLANDS
Las Palmas
IAMAT Coord., Calvo Viera, MD
Tel. 350 071

CAYMAN ISLANDS
Grand Cayman
IAMAT Center
Tel. 949 7400

CHILE
Santiago
Clinicas las Condes
Tel. 211 1002

CHINA
Beijing
Beijing Emergency Center
Tel. 33 2558
Shanghai
Zhong Shan Hospital
Tel. 310 400

COLOMBIA
Barranquilla
IAMAT Center
Tel. 359 072

Bogota
Clinica Marly
  Tel. 287 1020
Cartagena
IAMAT Coord., Hernando
  Espinosa P., MD
  Tel. 51 775
Medellin
IAMAT Center
  Tel. 251 5639

COSTA RICA
San Jose
Clinica Americana
  Tel. 22 10 10

CURACAO
Willemstad
St. Elisabeth Hospital
  Tel. 25 100

CYPRUS
Nicosia
The Nicosia Clinic
  Tel. 77 022/3

DENMARK
Copenhagen
IAMAT Center
  Tel. 38 78 28

DJIBOUTI
Djibouti
IAMAT Coord., Guenael Rodier,
  MD
  Tel. 35 13 30

DOMINICAN REPUBLIC
Santiago
Clinica Corominas
  Tel. 582 1171
Santo Domingo
IAMAT Coord., Jose H. Ornes,
  MD
  Tel. 682 0171

EQUADOR
Quito
Luis Garrido Fuenzalida, MD
  Tel. 234 117

EGYPT
Cairo
IAMAT Center
  Tel. 910 816

EL SALVADOR
San Salvador
IAMAT Coord., Luis J. Escalante,
  MD
  Tel. 230 609

ENGLAND
London
IAMAT Center
  Tel. 235 5995

ETHIOPIA
Addis Ababa
IAMAT Coord., Guenet Kifle, MD
  Tel. 443 242

FIJI
Suva
IAMAT Coord., Robin Mitchell,
  MBBS
  Tel. 36 1131

FINLAND
Helsinki
IAMAT Coord., Martin von
  Bonsdorff, MD
  Tel. 636 377

FRANCE
Cannes
IAMAT Center
  Tel. 68 27 28
Nice
IAMAT Center
  Tel. 88 61 64

GABON
Lambarene
Albert Schweitzer Hospital

GAMBIA
Banjul
IAMAT Center
  Tel. Banjul 81118

GERMANY
Bonn
Medizinische Universitaetsklinik
Tel. 280 2256
Hamburg
IAMAT Coord., Gerhard
Brockmann, MD
Tel. 479 919
Heidelberg
Medizinische Universitaetsklinik
Prof. G. Schettler, MD
Tel. 564 791
Munich
IAMAT Coord., Arnulf Borchers,
MD
Tel. 646 239

GHANA
Accra
Tudu Clinic
Tel. 24 833

GREECE
Athens
IAMAT Coord., Panayiotis
Babilis, MD
Tel. 652 9003
Rhodes
IAMAT Coord., John E. Sotiriou,
MD
Tel. 30 455

GRENADA
St. George's
IAMAT Coord., Bernard E.
Gittens, MBBS
Tel. 4380

GUADELOUPE
Pointe-A-Pitre
IAMAT Coord., Georges Nithila,
MD
Tel. 820 166

GUATEMALA
Guatemala
Hospital Herrera Lierandi
Tel. 66 771

GUINEA
Conakry
IAMAT Coord., Mamadou S.
Diallo, MD
Tel. 461 326

GUINEA-BISSAU
Bissau
IAMAT Coord., Kassem
Dahrouge, MD
Tel. 21 52 02

GUYANA
Georgetown
St. Joseph's Mercy Hospital
Tel. 72 070

HAITI
Port-Au-Prince
Hospital du Canape Vert
Tel. 21 052

HONDURAS
Tegucigalpa
IAMAT Coord., Eva Mannheim
de Gomez, MD
Tel. 321 023

HONG KONG
Hong Kong
IAMAT Coord., Patrick Ko, MD
Tel. (5) 265 131

HUNGARY
Budapest
IAMAT Coord., Istvan Lang, MD
Tel. 767 921

ICELAND
Reykjavik
St. Joseph's Hospital
Tel. 19 600

INDIA
Bombay
IAMAT Coord., R. H. Dastur, MD
Tel. 822 5638
Calcutta
Belle Vue Clinic

Tel. 442 321
Madras
H.M. Hospital
Tel. 72 236
New Delhi
IAMAT Coord., Harish Khosla,
MBBS
Tel. 312 351

INDONESIA
Jakarta
IAMAT Center
Tel. 714 591

IRAN
Teheran
IAMAT Coord., Gholam Ali
Nasseh, MD
Tel. 281 374

IRELAND, NORTHERN
Belfast
IAMAT Coord., Patrick T.
McGeough, MD
Tel. 777 759

IRELAND, REPUBLIC OF
Dublin
IAMAT Coord., John F.
Fleetwood, MD
Tel. 972 727

ISRAEL
Haifa
IAMAT Coord., G. Almagor, MD
Tel. (065) 66 274
Jerusalem
IAMAT Coord., Meir Litman, MD
Tel. 818 925
Tel Aviv
IAMAT Coord., Victor Zaigraeff,
MD
Tel. 251 095

ITALY
Bologna
IAMAT Coord., Frederick
Caronna, MD
Tel. 274 516

Florence
IAMAT Coord., Carlo Smorlesi,
MD
Tel. 475 411
Milan
IAMAT Coord., Bettina Sturlese,
MD
Tel. 805 7831
Naples
IAMAT Coord., Tommaso
Patarino, MD
Tel. 324 728
Palermo
IAMAT Coord., Louis J. Pepe, MD
Tel. 572 540
Rome
IAMAT Coord., Luigi Cardi, MD
Tel. 861 434
Venice
IAMAT Coord., Salvatore
Saccardo, MD
Tel. 522 1370

JAMAICA
Kingston
IAMAT Coord., George P. Provan,
MD
Tel. 927 8069
Montego Bay
IAMAT Coord., Alvin Lue, MD
Tel. 952 5833

JAPAN
Kyoto
Yoshio Sakabe, MD
Tel. 231 1624
Tokyo
Tokyo Hospital
Tel. 392 6151

JORDAN
Amman
IAMAT Coord., Z.A. Malhas, MD
Tel. 671 177

KENYA
Nairobi
IAMAT Coord., Manuel J. D'Cruz,
MB

Tel. 61 563
(Note: In Nairobi, IAMAT
members planning a safari in
East Africa may obtain a tourist
membership for $3.50 from the
Flying Doctors' Society of
Africa which offers ambulance
flights in emergencies.
Flying Doctors' Society of Africa
P.O. Box 30125, Nairobi
Tel. 501 301)

KOREA
Seoul
Kangnam St. Mary's Hospital
Tel. 593 9121

KUWAIT
Kuwait
Mowasat Hospital
Tel. 611 536

LAOS
Vientiane
IAMAT Coord., Prof. Vannareth
Raipho, MD
Tel. 2590

LEBANON
Beirut
IAMAT Coord., Jean Moadie, MD
Tel. 343 631
American University of Beirut
Hospital
Tel. 340 460

LESOTHO
Maseru
IAMAT Coord., Strong Thabo
Makenete, MD
Tel. 312 292

LUXEMBOURG
Luxembourg
IAMAT Coord., R. Schaus, MD
Tel. 489 268

MACAO
Macao
IAMAT Coord., L.C. Chiu, MD
Tel. 2590

MADEIRA
Funchal
IAMAT Center
Tel. 42 227

MADAGASCAR
Antananarivo
IAMAT Center
Tel. 268 62

MALAWI
Blantyre
Malamulo Hospital
Tel. 636 999

MALI
Bamako
IAMAT Coord., Daouda Keita,
MD
Tel. 22 41 37

MALAYSIA
Kuala Lumpur
Goh Tuck Keong, MD
Tel. 423 773

MALTA
Msida
IAMAT Coord., Robert Naudi,
MD
Tel. 332 739

MARTINIQUE
Fort-De-France
IAMAT Coord., Raymond
Rosenfeld, MD
Tel. 716 502

MAURITIUS
Port Louis
IAMAT Coord., M. Ibrahim
Joomun, MD
Tel. 085 934

MEXICO
Acapulco
IAMAT Coord., Francisco Mora
B., MD
Tel. 39 443
Cancun
IAMAT Coord., Jose Alba V., MD

Tel. 41 682
Mexico City
IAMAT Coord., Prof. Francisco
  Biagi, MD
  Tel. 524 9640
Oaxaca
Horacio Tenorio S., MD
  Tel. 66 285
Puerto Vallarta
IAMAT Coord., John H. Mabrey,
  MD
  Tel. 22 849
Taxco
IAMAT Coord., C. Garcia Torres,
  MD
  Tel. 20 567

MONGOLIA
Ulan Bator
Republic's Special Polyclinic
  Tel. 54 236

MOROCCO
Rabat
H. Moystad, MD
  Tel. 80 243

NEPAL
Kathmandu
Medical Clinic
  Tel. 211 213

THE NETHERLANDS
Amsterdam
IAMAT Center
  Tel. 626 886
The Hague
IAMAT Center
  Tel. 466 466

NEW ZEALAND
Auckland
IAMAT Coord., Lan Johnson, MB
  Tel. 505 060
Wellington
IAMAT Coord., Harold Haydon
  Gray, MD
  Tel. 862 124

NICARAGUA
Managua
Clinica Tiscapa
  Tel. 71 300

NIGERIA
Lagos
IAMAT Coord., Bimbola
  Ogunkelu, MD
  Tel. 962 242

NORWAY
Oslo
IAMAT Coord., Ornulf Jaer, MD
  Tel. 530 796

PAKISTAN
Islamabad
IAMAT Center
  821 458
Lahore
IAMAT Center
  Tel. 881 454

PANAMA
Colon
Clemente P. Garnes, MD
  Tel. 471 780
Panama
IAMAT Center
  Tel. 230 464

PAPUA NEW GUINEA
Boroko
IAMAT Coord., James E. Jacobi,
  MD
  Tel. 255 932

PERU
Lima
IAMAT Coord., Juan E. Dyer, MD
  Tel. 417 946
British American Hospital
  Tel. 403 570

PARAGUAY
Asuncion
IAMAT Coord., M. Gonzalez
  Oddone, MD
  Tel. 200 471

PHILIPPINES
Manila
IAMAT Coord., Juan G. Bailon, MD
Tel. 877 720

PORTUGAL
Lisbon
IAMAT Coord., David Ernst, MB
Tel. 554 113

QATAR
Doha
IAMAT Coord., S. Ahmad Kalantar, MD
Tel. 324 514

RWANDA
Kigali
IAMAT Center
Tel. 56 77

SAUDI ARABIA
Riyadh
IAMAT Coord., Ibrahim Fawzy, MD
Tel. 464 8116

SCOTLAND
Glasgow
IAMAT Coord., Nathaniel Chazan, MB
Tel. 554 2989

SENEGAL
Dakar
IAMAT Coord., Louis LeBlanc, MD
Tel. 21 35 93

SIERRA LEONE
Freetown
IAMAT Coord., J. Holst-Roness, MB
Tel. 26 671

SINGAPORE
Singapore
Youngberg Memorial Hospital
Tel. 285 2555

SOMALIA
Mogadishu
IAMAT Coord., Ali Salah Abdi, MD
21 447

SOUTH AFRICA
Johannesburg
IAMAT Coord., Joseph Teeger, MB
Tel. 728 4298

SPAIN
Barcelona
IAMAT Coord., M. Dianne McCarthy, MD
Tel. 200 2924
Madrid
IAMAT Coord., Enrique Puerta Scott, MD
Tel. 234 5811
Unidad Medica Anglo-Americana
Tel. 431 2229

SRI LANKA
Colombo
IAMAT Coord., M.P. Kanthi Kirtisinghe, MB
Tel. 573 957

SUDAN
Khartoum
W. Williams, MD
Tel. 44 479

SURINAME
Paramaribo
IAMAT Coord., F.J.C. Fung A. Foek, MD
Tel. 99 158

SWAZILAND
Mbabane
Mbabane Clinic Services
Tel. 24 25/6

SWEDEN
Goteborg
IAMAT Coord., Sven Erik Hyllner, MD

Tel. 117 914
Malmo
IAMAT Coord., Claus Garmer,
MD
Tel. 16 0312
Stockholm
IAMAT Coord., Olle Norrbohm,
MD
Tel. 768 5859

SWITZERLAND
Basel
IAMAT Coord., Martin Eisner,
MD
Tel. 234 934
Bern
IAMAT Coord., Prof. Ed.
Maibach, MD
Tel. 252 040
Geneva
IAMAT Coord., Nicolas
Petitpierre, MD
Tel. 312 204
Zurich
IAMAT Coord., Beat A. Gurtler,
MD
Tel. 724 1444

SYRIA
Damascus
IAMAT Coord., Faissal Kanan,
MD
Tel. 719 850

TAIWAN
Taipei
Taiwan Adventist Hospital
Tel. 771 8151

TANZANIA
Serengeti National Park
(See *Kenya* for information on
Flying Doctors' Society of
Africa)

THAILAND
Bangkok
Bangkok Adventist Hospital
Tel. 281 1422

TRINIDAD
Port of Spain
IAMAT Coord., Gordon A. Toby,
MD
Tel. 622 2544

TUNISIA
Tunis
IAMAT Coord., Ahmed Zribi, MD
Tel. 286 871

TURKEY
Ankara
IAMAT Coord., Osman Coskun,
MD
Tel. 295 764
Istanbul
IAMAT Coord., Ozkan Duygun,
MD
Tel. 357 4156

UGANDA
Kampala
IAMAT Coord., Mukhtar Ahmad,
MBBS
Tel. 231 137

UNITED ARAB EMIRATES
Abu Dhabi
IAMAT Coord., Salem F Al-
Damluji, MD
Tel. 338 428

URUGUAY
Montevideo
Hospital Britanico
Tel. 800 020

VENEZUELA
Caracas
IAMAT Coord., Nissim M.
Abecasis S., MD
Tel. 529 603

YUGOSLAVIA
Belgrade
IAMAT Coord., L. Petronijevic,
MD
Tel. 451 308

Duprovnik
IAMAT Coord., Josip Rehak, MD
Tel. 22 677

ZAIRE
Kinshasa
IAMAT Coord., A.C. Jain,, MBBS
Tel. 26 551

ZAMBIA
Lusaka
IAMAT Coord., Chifumbe
Chintu, MD
Tel. 253 438

ZIMBABWE
Harare
IAMAT Coord., J. Arthur
Matenga, MB
Tel. 882 750

IV
INDICES

1. INDEX OF COUNTRIES

Finland	2	**J**	
France	2	Jamaica	4
French Guiana	7	Japan	16
French Polynesia	22	Jordan	9

G

		K	
Gabon	18	Kampuchea	13
Gambia	18	Kenya	17
Germany (East)	2	Kiribati	22
Germany (West)	2	Korea	16
Ghana	18	Kuwait	9
Gibraltar	2		
Great Britain	2	**L**	
Greece	3	Laos	13
Greenland	2	Lebanon	10
Grenada	4	Lesotho	21
Guadeloupe	4	Liberia	18
Guam	22	Libya	9
Guatemala	6	Luxembourg	2
Guinea	19		
Guinea-Bissau	18	**M**	
Guyana	7	Macao	16
		Madagascar	20
H		Madeira	4
Haiti	6	Malawi	20
Honduras	6	Malaysia	14
Hong Kong	16	Maldives	15
Hungary	2	Mali	19
		Malta	3
I		Martinique	4
Iceland	2	Mauritania	18
India	13	Mauritius	4
Indonesia	14	Mexico	5
Iran	10	Mongolia	16
Iraq	11	Morocco	9
Ireland	2	Mozambique	20
Israel	9		
Italy	2	**N**	
Ivory Coast	19	Namibia	20

Nauru	22	Sao Tome	19
Nepal	15	Saudi Arabia	11
Netherlands	2	Senegal	18
New Caledonia	22	Seychelles	16
New Guinea	23	Sierra Leone	19
New Hebrides	23	Singapore	15
New Zealand	23	Solomon Is.	23
Nicaragua	6	Somalia	17
Niger	18	South Africa	21
Nigeria	18	Spain	2
Niue	22	Sri Lanka	15
Norway	2	St. Helena	3
		St. Kitts	4

O

Oman	11	St. Lucia	4
		St. Martin	4

P

		St. Pierre	3
Pacific Is. (U.S.)	22	St. Vincent	4
Pakistan	12	Sudan	17
Panama	7	Suriname	7
Papua	23	Swaziland	20
Paraguay	6	Sweden	2
Peru	8	Switzerland	2
Philippines	16	Syria	10
Pitcairn Is.	22		
Poland	2		
Portugal	2	**T**	
Puerto Rico	3	Tahiti	22

Q

		Taiwan	15
Qatar	11	Tanzania	17
		Thailand	14
		Tobago	4
R		Togo	18
Reunion	4	Tonga	22
Romania	2	Trinidad	4
Russia	2	Tunisia	9
Rwanda	17	Tuvalu	22
		Turkey	2

S

		U	
Samoa (American)	22	Uganda	17
Samoa (Western)	22	U.S.A.	2

For other details, consult
the Table of Contents

2. SUBJECT INDEX

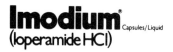

Imodium® Capsules/Liquid
(loperamide HCl)

DESCRIPTION: IMODIUM (loperamide hydrochloride), 4-(p-chlorophenyl)-4-hydroxy-N,N-dimethyl-α,α-diphenyl-1-piperidinebutyramide monohydrochloride, is a synthetic antidiarrheal for oral use.

IMODIUM is available in 2 mg capsules and as a liquid containing 1 mg / 5 ml.

The inactive ingredients are:
in capsules: Lactose, magnesium stearate, starch, and talc.
in liquid: Alcohol, artificial anise flavor, artificial cherry flavor, citric acid monohydrate, glycerin, methylparaben, and propylparaben.

CLINICAL PHARMACOLOGY: *In vitro* and animal studies show that IMODIUM acts by slowing intestinal motility and by affecting water and electrolyte movement through the bowel. IMODIUM inhibits peristaltic activity by a direct effect on the circular and longitudinal muscles of the intestinal wall.

In man, IMODIUM prolongs the transit time of the intestinal contents. It reduces the daily fecal volume, increases the viscosity and bulk density, and diminishes the loss of fluid and electrolytes. Tolerance to the antidiarrheal effect has not been observed.

Clinical studies have indicated that the apparent elimination half-life of loperamide in man is 10.8 hours with a range of 9.1-14.4 hours. Plasma levels of unchanged drug remain below 2 nanograms per ml after the intake of a 2 mg capsule of IMODIUM. Plasma levels are highest approximately five hours after administration of the capsule and 2.5 hours after the liquid. The peak plasma levels of loperamide were similar for both formulations. Of the total excreted in urine and feces, most of the administered drug was excreted in feces.

In those patients in whom biochemical and hematological parameters were monitored during clinical trials, no trends toward abnormality during IMODIUM therapy were noted. Similarly, urinalyses, EKG and clinical ophthalmological examinations did not show trends toward abnormality.

INDICATIONS AND USAGE: IMODIUM is indicated for the control and symptomatic relief of acute nonspecific diarrhea and of chronic diarrhea associated with inflammatory bowel disease. IMODIUM is also indicated for reducing the volume of discharge from ileostomies.

CONTRAINDICATIONS: IMODIUM is contraindicated in patients with known hypersensitivity to the drug and in those in whom constipation must be avoided.

WARNINGS: IMODIUM should not be used in the case of acute dysentery, which is characterized by blood in stools and elevated temperatures.

Fluid and electrolyte depletion may occur in patients who have diarrhea. The use of IMODIUM does not preclude the administration of appropriate fluid and electrolyte therapy.

In some patients with acute ulcerative colitis, and in pseudomembranous colitis associated with broad-spectrum antibiotics, agents which inhibit intestinal motility or delay intestinal transit time have been reported to induce toxic megacolon. IMODIUM therapy should be discontinued promptly if abdominal distention occurs or if other untoward symptoms develop in patients with acute ulcerative colitis.

IMODIUM should be used with special caution in young children because of the greater variability of response in this age group. Dehydration, particularly in younger children, may further influence the variability of response to IMODIUM.

PRECAUTIONS:
General: In acute diarrhea, if clinical improvement is not observed in 48 hours, the administration of IMODIUM should be discontinued.

Patients with hepatic dysfunction should be monitored closely for signs of CNS toxicity because of the apparent large first pass biotransformation.

Information for Patients: Patients should be advised to check with their physician if their diarrhea doesn't stop after a few days or if they develop a fever.

Drug Interactions: There was no evidence in clinical trials of drug interactions with concurrent medications.

Carcinogenesis, mutagenesis, impairment of fertility: In an 18-month rat study with doses up to 133 times the maximum human dose (on a mg/kg basis), there was no evidence of carcinogenesis. Mutagenicity studies were not conducted. Reproduction studies in rats indicated that high doses (150-200 times the human dose) could cause marked female infertility and reduced male fertility.

Pregnancy – Teratogenic Effects – Pregnancy Category B: Reproduction studies in rats and rabbits have revealed no evidence of impaired fertility or harm to the fetus at doses up to 30 times the human dose. Higher doses impaired the survival of mothers and nursing young. The studies offered no evidence of teratogenic activity. There are, however, no adequate and well controlled studies in pregnant women. Because animal reproduction studies are not always predictive of human response, this drug should be used during pregnancy only if clearly needed.

Nursing Mothers: It is not known whether this drug is excreted in human milk. Because many drugs are excreted in human milk, caution should be exercised when IMODIUM is administered to a nursing woman.

Pediatric Use: See the "Warnings" Section for information on the greater variability of response in this age group.

In case of accidental overdosage of IMODIUM by children, see "Overdosage" Section for suggested treatment.

ADVERSE REACTIONS: The adverse effects reported during clinical investigations of IMODIUM are difficult to distinguish from symptoms associated with the diarrheal syndrome. Adverse experiences recorded during clinical studies with IMODIUM were generally of a minor and self-limiting nature. They were more commonly observed during the treatment of chronic diarrhea.

The following patient complaints have been reported and are listed in decreasing order of frequency with the exception of hypersensitivity reactions which is listed first since it may be the most serious.

- Hypersensitivity reactions (including skin rash) have been reported with IMODIUM use.
- Abdominal pain, distention or discomfort
- Nausea and vomiting
- Constipation
- Tiredness
- Drowsiness or dizziness
- Dry mouth

DRUG ABUSE AND DEPENDENCE:

Abuse: A specific clinical study designed to assess the abuse potential of loperamide at high doses resulted in a finding of extremely low abuse potential. Additionally, after years of extensive use there has been no evidence of abuse or dependence.

Dependence: Physical dependence to IMODIUM in humans has not been observed. However, studies in morphine-dependent monkeys demonstrated that loperamide hydrochloride at doses above those recommended for humans prevented signs of morphine withdrawal. However, in humans, the naloxone challenge pupil test, which when positive indicates opiate-like effects, performed after a single high dose, or after more than two years of therapeutic use of IMODIUM, was negative. Orally administered IMODIUM (loperamide formulated with magnesium stearate) is both highly insoluble and penetrates the CNS poorly.

OVERDOSAGE: Animal pharmacological and toxicological data indicate that overdosage in man may result in constipation, CNS depression and gastrointestinal irritation. Clinical trials have demonstrated that a slurry of activated charcoal administered promptly after ingestion of loperamide hydrochloride can reduce the amount of drug which is absorbed into the systemic circulation by as much as ninefold. If vomiting occurs spontaneously upon ingestion, a slurry of 100 gms of activated charcoal should be administered orally as soon as fluids can be retained.

If vomiting has not occurred, gastric lavage should be performed followed by administration of 100 gms of the activated charcoal slurry through the gastric tube. In the event of overdosage, patients should be monitored for signs of CNS depression for at least 24 hours. Children may be more sensitive to central nervous system effects than adults. If CNS depression is observed, naloxone may be administered. If responsive to naloxone, vital signs must be monitored carefully for recurrence of symptoms of drug overdose for at least 24 hours after the last dose of naloxone.

In view of the prolonged action of loperamide and the short duration (one to three hours) of naloxone, the patient must be monitored closely and treated repeatedly with naloxone as indicated. Since relatively little drug is excreted in the urine, forced diuresis is not expected to be effective for IMODIUM overdosage.

In clinical trials an adult who took three 20 mg doses within a 24 hour period was nauseated after the second dose and vomited after the third dose. In studies designed to examine the potential for side effects, intentional ingestion of up to 60 mg of loperamide hydrochloride in a single dose to healthy subjects resulted in no significant adverse effects.

DOSAGE AND ADMINISTRATION: (1 teaspoonful — 1 mg.; 1 capsule — 2 mg.)

Acute Diarrhea

Adults: The recommended initial dose is two IMODIUM Capsules or four teaspoonfuls of IMODIUM Liquid (4 mg) followed by one capsule or two teaspoonfuls of liquid (2 mg) after each unformed stool. Daily dosage should not exceed eight capsules or sixteen teaspoonfuls of liquid (16 mg). Clinical improvement is usually observed within 48 hours.

Children: IMODIUM use is not recommended for children under 2 years of age. In children 2 to 5 years of age (20 kg or less), IMODIUM Liquid should be used; for ages 6 to 12, either IMODIUM Liquid or Capsules may be used. For children 2 to 12 years of age, the following schedule for capsules or liquid will usually fulfill initial dosage requirements:

Recommended First Day Dosage Schedule

Two to five years: (13 to 20 kg)	1 mg t.i.d. (3 mg daily dose) (1 teaspoonful t.i.d.)
Five to eight years: (20 to 30 kg)	2 mg b.i.d. (4 mg daily dose) (2 teaspoonfuls or 1 capsule b.i.d.)
Eight to twelve years: (greater than 30 kg)	2 mg t.i.d. (6 mg daily dose) (2 teaspoonfuls or 1 capsule t.i.d.)

Recommended Subsequent Daily Dosage

Following the first treatment day, it is recommended that subsequent IMODIUM doses (1 mg / 10 kg body weight) be administered only after a loose stool. Total daily dosage should not exceed recommended dosages for the first day.

Chronic Diarrhea

Children: Although IMODIUM has been studied in a limited number of children with chronic diarrhea, the therapeutic dose for the treatment of chronic diarrhea in a pediatric population has not been established.

Adults: The recommended initial dose is two IMODIUM Capsules or four teaspoonfuls of IMODIUM Liquid (4 mg) followed by one capsule or two teaspoonfuls of liquid (2 mg) after each unformed stool until diarrhea is controlled, after which the dosage of IMODIUM should be reduced to meet individual requirements. When the optimal daily dosage has been established, this amount may then be administered as a single dose or in divided doses.

The average daily maintenance dosage in clinical trials was 4 to 8 mg (two to four capsules or four to eight teaspoonfuls of liquid). A dosage of 16 mg (eight capsules or sixteen teaspoonfuls of liquid) was rarely exceeded. If clinical improvement is not observed after treatment with 16 mg per day for at least 10 days, symptoms are unlikely to be controlled by further administration. IMODIUM administration may be continued if diarrhea cannot be adequately controlled with diet or specific treatment.

HOW SUPPLIED: Liquid – containing 1 mg loperamide hydrochloride per 5 ml. Bottles of 4 oz.

Capsules – each capsule contains 2 mg of loperamide hydrochloride. The capsules have a light green body and a dark green cap with "JANSSEN" imprinted on one segment and "IMODIUM" on the other segment. IMODIUM capsules are supplied in bottles of 100 and 500 and in blister packs of 10 × 10 capsules.

NDC 50458-410-04 (4 oz. Liquid)   **NDC** 50458-400-10 (100 capsules)
NDC 50458-400-01 (10 × 10 capsules – blister)   **NDC** 50458-400-50 (500 capsules)

Revised July 1985, January 1987

CAUTION: FEDERAL LAW PROHIBITS DISPENSING WITHOUT A PRESCRIPTION

An original product of   JANSSEN PHARMACEUTICA INC.
JANSSEN PHARMACEUTICA, n.v.   Piscataway, NJ 08854
B-2340 Beerse, Belgium   U.S. Patent 3,714,159

world leader in antidiarrheal research

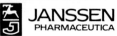

JANSSEN
PHARMACEUTICA

Piscataway, NJ 08854

1P41K00F-M